Dieter Roth

Museum of Contemporary Art, Chicago

Preface

By Mary Jane Jacob, *Chief Curator*

At a moment when the art world appears concerned with identifying new "stars" and charting escalating market prices, it is interesting, though not fashionable, to focus on an artist whose distance from the commercial art scene, dedication to making affordable, mass-produced books, and experimentation with unconventional, unstable, sometimes even biodegradable materials have been his paramount concerns. An enigmatic figure whose disinterest in public exposure has made him less well known than other major artists of his generation, Dieter Roth has maintained a sense of experimentation and rebellion in his art for more than 30 years. Roth is probably best known for his artists' books, a field in which he is the foremost figure and highly influential. Through his use of design, language, and materials, he has done more than any other artist to reinterpret the book as a concept.

It is most appropriate that the Museum of Contemporary Art sponsor this exhibition of Dieter Roth as its first one-person show of a book artist. During its recent history the Museum has been active in the area of artists' books, periodicals, and records by collecting these materials, beginning in 1979, through the support of the Men's Council. Subsequently, an ongoing program has been established to add to and maintain this collection, which totals at present nearly 1300 titles and includes, in virtually all cases, duplicate copies of each item for archival as well as display purposes. While the Museum has almost continuously exhibited artists' books as part of installations of selected works from the collection and exhibitions, such as "Earthart from the Permanent Collection" in 1983, this is the first occasion that a book artist has been the subject of a special exhibition.

Exhibitions of Roth's work have been exceedingly rare in Europe and almost nonexistent in the United States. We are extremely fortunate that the artist's work is unusually well represented in Chicago by the collection of Ira G. Wool, and it is through the cooperation of Dr. Wool, a longtime friend of the artist, that it has been possible for the Museum of Contemporary Art to undertake this showing. In addition to books, Roth also creates paintings, sculptures, drawings, graphics, films, video, and installations; the explosive creativity and intensity which he brings to his work necessitates that these many avenues be explored simultaneously, and this is reflected in the scope of this exhibition. The Wool collection contains a near-complete set of Roth's publications, with unique items such as book covers and the 31-volume work *Collection of Flat Waste 1982*. In addition, a major chocolate painting, rubberband painting, palette paintings, glue paintings, and a special installation work, the *Chicago Wandbild,* are among the collection's highlights. For the loans of these works as well as altered postcards, drawings, sculptural works, and prints, and for his helpfulness throughout the organization of this exhibition, we are deeply indebted to Dr. Wool. Roth is also represented in Chicago in the extraordinary Neumann Family Collection. We would like to thank Mr. and Mrs. Morton G. Neumann for their willingness to lend their important collage with chocolate. The Museum of Contemporary Art's own artists' book collection has also been a major resource, and we are pleased to announce that with this exhibition the Museum has acquired about 100 books and 20 record albums as a gift of the artist – works which not only find an important place in the current show, but greatly enrich our collection, making it one of the finest in the country today.

For his generosity and efforts in preparing a film installation (previously undertaken at the Venice Biennale in 1982), which he has re-created especially for the Museum's Manilow Gallery, we would like to express our sincerest gratitude to Dieter Roth. His energy and enthusiasm have made this historical review of his directions over the last three decades an exciting event.

I would like also to thank Björn Roth who traveled from Iceland to assist his father, and Dennis O'Shea, Museum Technician, who played an essential role in facilitating the film project, as well as the other video and audio components of the exhibition. This publication will be an important means of presenting Roth's work to American audiences. For her contribution to this aspect of the exhibition, I would like especially to thank Ann Goldstein, whose insightful and intelligent essay follows; special thanks also are due to Mitzi B. Sabato who compiled the bibliography and assisted with the other phases of this exhibition, Terry Ann R. Neff who edited the catalogue, and Michael Glass who designed it. Finally, I would like to thank the Museum's Exhibition Committee, Men's Council, and Board of Trustees whose understanding of the unusual forms, unorthodox aesthetic, and unconventional means that permeate Roth's oeuvre, have made possible this exhibition.

Dieter Roth

By Ann Goldstein

The collection of Dr. Ira G. Wool is the result of an unusual collaboration between two friends, an artist and a collector (see fig. 1). Wool, a professor in biochemistry at the University of Chicago, met Roth in Berlin in 1971, through a scientist friend who took him to Oswald Wiener's restaurant/bar, "Exil." Wiener, along with fellow Viennese artists Günter Brus, Hermann Nitsch, Otto Mühl, and Rudolf Schwarzkogler, was exiled from Vienna for politically confrontational and degrading art performances. His Berlin bar became a meeting place for artists, including Dieter Roth. Ira Wool recalled:

> I was introduced to the man sitting next to me at Oswald's table one night, and I recognized the name. At the time, Dieter was not known in the United States, although I had heard of him through the Petersburg Press, where he had published prints. He was pleased that I had heard of him, and although he is generally rather reserved in meeting new people, he talked with me quite warmly. It was a phenomenal experience.[1]

Initially, Wool began collecting Roth's drawings and paintings. Subsequently, he met concrete poet Hansjörg Mayer, Roth's publisher and partner in Edition Hansjörg Mayer, through whom he became acquainted with and began to acquire Roth's artists' books as well as the other books published by this press.

> The first artists' book I ever saw, although I didn't consider it so at the time, was a notebook of Dieter's – one of his year's diaries – which he pulled out to show me one night. Its pages were filled with notes and drawings. It was the first thing of its kind I had ever seen. The diaries are unique works and are kept in Dieter's archives. Most of what I know of artists' books I learned from Dieter. The first artists' book I ever owned was Volume 20 in his *Collected Works,* a catalogue of a Berlin exhibition of Dieter's books and prints. The show opened during my year in Berlin, and in fact, Dieter invited me to the opening, scrawling the date, place, and time on a paper napkin. The show featured his books suspended by chains from the ceiling, and I must say I wasn't terribly impressed with them at the time. I remember saying to him that I thought the prints were great and that the reproductions in the catalogue and in the books were not very good. I didn't understand that the reproductions in the catalogue and in the books were exactly the way he wanted them: not very good.[2]

Soon, artists' books by Roth and many others filled Wool's library shelves – a historically significant collection, including many seminal and now rare works from the Fluxus artists as well as a recent addition by the late Marcel Broodthaers: a total collection approaching 1000 titles.

Ira Wool approaches his dual relationship with Roth – as friend and collector – with sensitivity and conscience. His commitment to Roth the artist is indicative of the responsibility that he assumes towards the creators of every artwork he collects. The friendship with Wool has brought Roth to Chicago, where he has left behind him a trail of artworks: hand-drawn books, drawings, paintings, and unfinished or ongoing works, including the *Chicago Wandbild,* begun in 1976. Friendship, nurtured by Roth's trust and Wool's uncompromising enthusiasm and commitment, has always taken precedence.

Fig. I.
Untitled (por. o. Ira), 1973. Pencil on paper.

D. Roth was born 46 years ago among the butchering Germans at that horrible stretch of time, when that cannibal, awful Hitler, Adolf, was just getting the Germans going at their best hit, butchering war. Hell was loose, but Roth survived, beatings and scoldings he survived, shitting and pissing in his timid pants, poor shaking little turd, he even managed to live through that rainstorm of bombs and grenades awful smashing horror, brought about on all, the living and the dead, by the horridly cruel cool English and the annihilatingly maneating cannibals, those fanty (fantastically) cruel citizens of the so-called United States of Northamerica, horrible mankillers. Roth got out of that place (described) by chance of being one of the citizens of his horrible home country, namely, selfrighteously, murderously Christian Switzerland. He survived, pantpissing there for 12 years. Then one of the friendly helped him out of it, getting to beautiful, beautiful Copenhagen. Having managed to happily survive there for a year, matrimony got him, catching up with him. An awfully, dreadfully fearful drain he fell down into, wriggling there, at the bottom, pissing in his wet pants, shitting and drinking terrible, awfully pissing lots, screaming for mercy. Again he managed to escape, this time to a place that soon proved to him to be full of his like, butchering bastards, dwellers in shit, pissing in their pissing wet pants, eating each others awful bodies and souls, dwellers of Hell. De did escape though, to another place, thoughtful eyes watching him (the eyes of his second parents, his children), doubling his raging shame. Steamer of the dampsteamingwet, shitpissing pants, stumbling around the corners of the all encompassing butcher's shop. Turdknickering awful bastard of fear, complaining (D.R., Barcelona, July 1976).[3]

Dieter Roth, a.k.a. **dieter roth, DITERROT, diter rot, Dietrich Roth, Karl-Dieterich Roth,** speaks best for himself, but beware: His words, gestures, and marks are seasoned with autobiographical license and mixed with experiments in typography, semiotics, and exotic substances. His oeuvre contains his chronology, each piece the unpredictable fusion of seemingly disparate parts and sources, a spiral: Roth awakening his deepest horrors, humors, and fantasies to meld into his elusive Tower of Babel.

Pouring one material into another, changing one style into another, combining one medium with another, Dieter Roth is the catalyst in a metamorphosis that breeds a multitude of forms: artists' books, paintings, poetry, graphics, sculpture, music, installations, letters, and postcards. In a dissolution of the boundaries separating art and life, Roth converges the organic with the social and the personal worlds into artforms that, too, are subject to life's processes – for example, his use of sour milk –

> I discovered the potential of sour milk by accident. It was at a special period in my life, when I was married in Iceland, – that I sneaked out at night to draw what you might call "dirty pictures." I was very ashamed of this bent and to destroy these pictures I once poured sour milk over them. Then I noticed that they became very beautiful. Subsequently I always pour sour milk over pictures that weren't beautiful or didn't work out. Sour milk is like landscape, ever changing. Works of art should be like that, – they should change like man himself, grow old and die.[4]

Change, the process of life, is at the essence of Roth's art – from the metabolism of the organic works to the subtle, delicate mirror image of a drawing transferred onto the preceding blank page in a bookwork and then reworked by Roth so that the new image will transfer back onto the original. The notion of double-sided works is most directly expressed in Roth's two-handed drawings, in which he uses both hands simultaneously to create a mirror-image composition (see fig. 2).

In his efforts to bring life into his art Roth draws upon the world and all of its physical and social precipitates, throwing them into unexpected contexts with an insistence on technical and conceptual control for every seeming imperfection he creates. These styles and processes are subsumed into Roth's pictorial and literal content, which centers around and extends from his existential individuality, his elusive humor, and his obsession for imperfection and bodily functions, where art is just another excretion.

> I don't work very hard at making perfect works of art. I'm not very keen on being the best or making perfect things. I often wait until I'm under the weather, ill, tired or hung over to make things. Making art is like making other things in life, it depends on your mood, your state of mind. You make good things and everything in between. But even then, when I try to create in this state of mind, my upbringing makes itself felt and I end up writing or painting well. It shows that I haven't managed to break loose from my youth. I'm afraid of showing the truth. I'm still a slave to something. We are all slaves to something.
>
> Life itself is slavery. You may talk as a free man and your words may be free, but your soul isn't.[5]

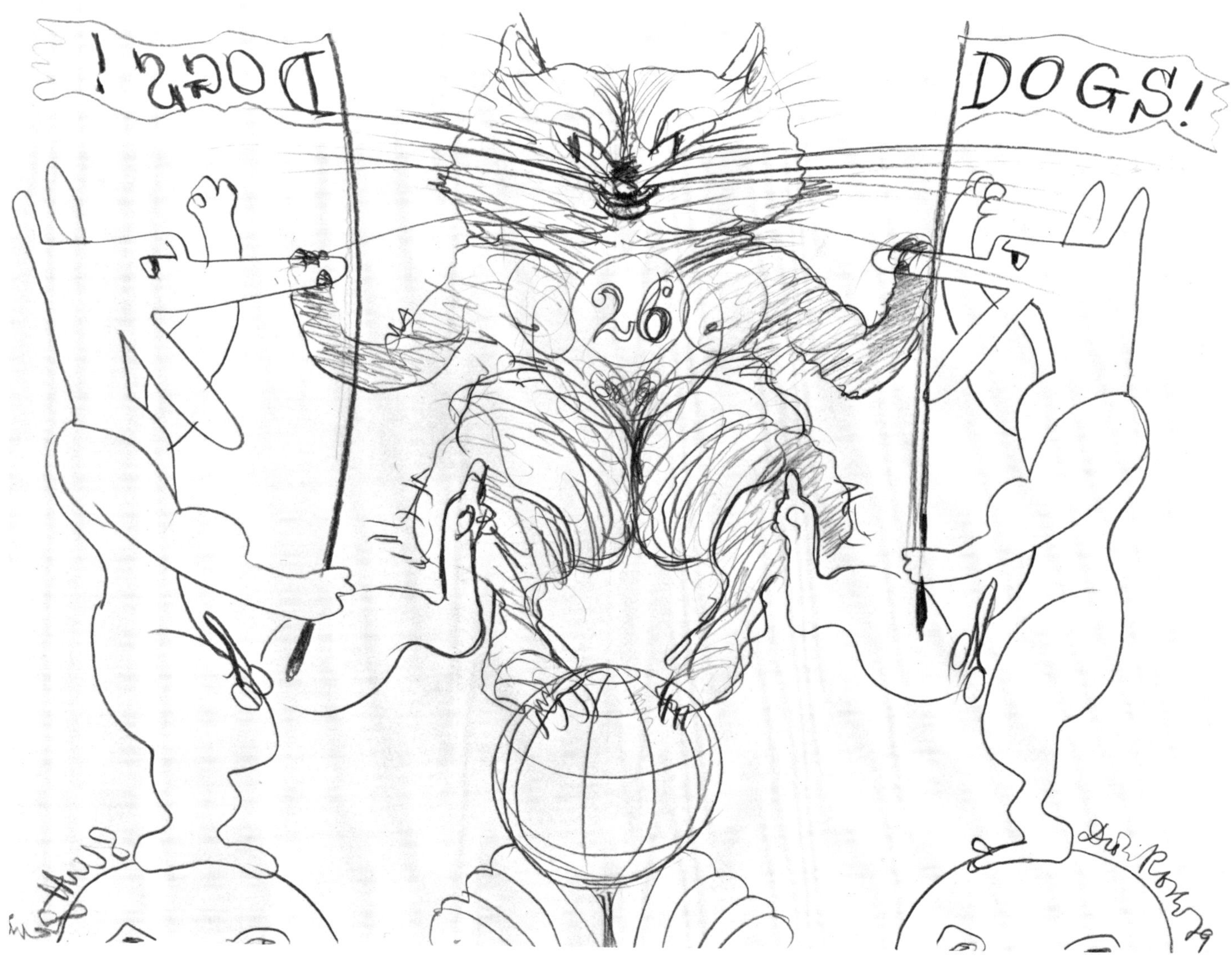

Dieter Roth was born in 1930 in Hanover, Germany, to a German mother and a Swiss father. World War II provided Roth with his first major relocation, and was the source of an indelible German anger and quest for exposition of the genocidal tendencies of the human character. In 1943 Roth and his brother were sent to Switzerland for safekeeping. Roth's brother was sent to Bucher (he later became a butcher), and Dieter was sent to a hotel for German refugees and dissidents in Zurich. During his four years in the hotel Roth went to school at the Gymnasium, studying Greek, Latin, and French. The soundproof rooms of the hotel provided a refuge for Jews and others escaping the Third Reich – a place to talk, yell, and perform – an inspiration to the young Roth.

Roth traces his first interest in art and literature to his boyhood in Germany, where he admired the paintings in galleries and tried to imitate the 18th-century Romantic poetry of Goethe and Schiller. The teenage Roth, lonely in his Swiss hotel room, began drawing pictures. He recalled: "I wanted to be an artist for the fame of it."[6]

Roth pursued his interest, extending his emotions into drawings, paintings, etchings, and poetry, and dropped out of the Gymnasium at the age of 17 to take a job as a graphic design apprentice in an advertising agency, while continuing to expand his personal work into lino- and woodcuts, collages, and lithographs.

Roth's unsuccessful attempt in 1950 to avoid military service was followed by a year of feigning insanity, and his dismissal from the army. In 1953 he published the first of his many collaborative efforts, an art review, *Spirale,* produced by Roth, concrete poet Eugen Gomringer, and painter Marcel Wyss as a vehicle to publish their own poems. Roth's poems were called kitsch and sentimental, and this negative reaction sent him to the Arles River, where he cast off onto the water a boat bearing the poems and some paintings. The experience left him with a writer's block that he claims lasted until he was 35 years old.

Nevertheless, his visual works continued growing in number of forms and substances. And Roth delighted in his increasing contacts with other artists. Through his friendship with Swiss artist Daniel Spoerri, which began in 1953, Roth became acquainted with other artists in French art critic Pierre Restany's Nouveau Réalisme group, and participated in the international Fluxus movement of the 1950s through the 1970s, collaborating with Spoerri, Robert Filliou, Nam June Paik, Charlotte Moorman, Dick Higgins, George Brecht, and Emmett Williams. Both art movements sought the dissolution of the boundaries separating art and life through their "events" and aesthetic confrontations. Roth shared this attitude, as is evident in his experiments in optical art, film, his first "baked" dough sculptures, and, in 1954, the completion of his first artists' book.

Fig. 2.
DOGS (26) from *2 times 5 DOGS* (22/100), 1979. Pencil on paper. Collection of Museum of Contemporary Art, Chicago.

The late 1950s through the 1960s was a period of extensive international travel and work. In 1956 Roth worked as a textile designer in Copenhagen; this was followed by marriage and a move to Reykjavík, Iceland, in 1957. In 1958 his first trip to the United States, at the invitation of Newcomb Montgomery, an American architect impressed by Roth's jewelry designs in Iceland, was for the purpose of teaching at the Philadelphia Museum College of Art. His arrival, with Swiss Constructivistic sketches in hand, was greeted with rejection (the school had just cast off its own resident Swiss Constructivist). A short stint as a visiting critic at Yale University, followed by four additional months of labor, finally gained Roth the fare for his return to Iceland.

In 1964 Roth came again to Philadelphia to accept an offer to produce work in the private press of a former teacher at the Philadelphia Museum College of Art. When Roth's host saw the artist's current messy, emotional products, bearing no resemblance to his pure, clean, concrete work of 1958, this offer also soured. Roth finally did teach (graphics) at the Philadelphia Museum and finished his book *Snow* on their presses.

The 1960s provided Roth with a number of teaching stints: a return to Yale in the School of Architecture in late 1964; Rhode Island School of Design, Providence, in 1965; and London's Watford School of Art and the Akademie in Düsseldorf in 1968. In his personal work he continued his material and media experiments and hybrids: pressings and squashings as graphics, etchings with chocolate and bananas, books with texts printed on plastic or foil, bags filled with glued, dyed cheese, lamb cutlets, etc., and self-portraits and sculpture made out of food. While in Düsseldorf Roth joined with Hansjörg Mayer (see fig. 3) as his partner in Edition Hansjörg Mayer to publish artists' books and audioworks.

Roth's inexhaustible, digestive expansion has continued through the 1970s into the 1980s: installations with rotting cheese, painting, drawing, audio and video works, collaborative efforts, and the perennial artists' books filled with everything from a single image xeroxed so many times that the image disappears, to plastic sleeves filling volumes with Roth's collected detritus. The biography can no longer catch up with Roth as he travels between his residences in Germany, Switzerland, and Iceland, leaving behind trails of art and poetry.

> It is a curious thing that the German temperament, which in other spheres so often insists on clearly polarized antitheses, none the less favours blurring over the particular demarcation line between literature and art.[7]

Dieter Roth continues this Germanic tradition, that recently stems from the Dada and Constructivist movements, but is traceable back to the Gutenberg Bible. From his pictorial experiments in concrete poetry to words in texts, the typographical element has been subject to Roth's manipulations. Most comprehensive has been the treatment of his own name, the subject of an ongoing typographical experiment in the expressive qualities of upper- versus lower-case letters and variations in spelling and signature.

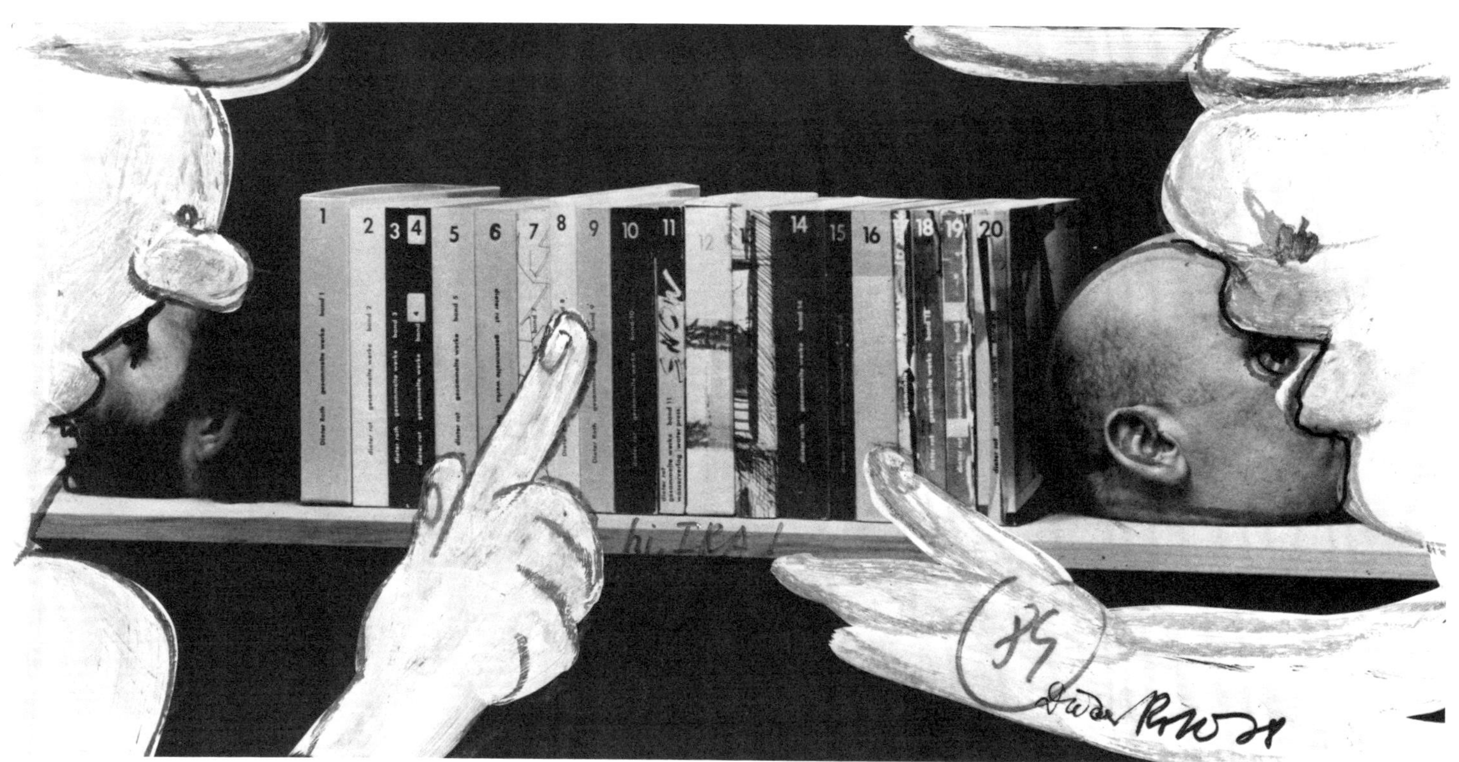

Fig. 3.
Untitled (hi, Ira!), 1978. Paint and oil pastel on photograph.

> The name is written all ways and consequently leads one to think that the products of the author may be regarded or read as different ones, – that even the same text, printed in different editions, has differed from itself in terms of time, that at least a sense of distance has crept into the text, which does not allow it to remain the same.[8]

It was **dieter roth** who, in 1953, first published his work in the Swiss periodical *Spirale.* In 1957, living in the austere, isolated environment of Iceland, **diter rot** experimented in the reductive, Minimalist approaches prevalent internationally at that time, as well as continuing the purist Swiss concrete style of geometrics and primary colors. Simplification is also a tool in German language and spelling – the reduction and deletion of what are considered to be unnecessary letters and sounds. And it was in the German language that **DITERROT** preferred to express himself in 1967, inviting confusion with the 18th-century French encyclopedist. The 1960s conclude with **dieter rot**'s signature on the first of his *Collected Works* series of artists' books, eventually conforming to the basic uniformity of **Dieter Roth**, but never so consistent as to be predictable, for he pulled out his given name, **Karl-Dietrich Roth**, or its slight abbreviation, **Dieterich Roth**, to sign his *scheisse* books, a series of collections and fragments of his poetry, in the mid-1970s.

Artists' books are nontraditional in nature, with the artist assuming and transcending the roles of author and illustrator and producing a work conceived, executed, and received in book form. In the 20th century, artists' books can be traced back to the typographical experiments of El Lissitsky's Constructivism and Futurist, Dada, and Surrealist publications.

Intimacy, the socio-political possibilities of the printed multiple, as well as artistic interests of the avant-garde, contributed to a surge in the production of artists' books beginning in the 1950s. The first group to take hold of this form was the international Fluxus movement of the 1950s through the 1970s. In Germany Fluxus artist Wolf Vostell published *dé-collage,* a periodical composed of contributions by various artists, with Vostell's term "dé-collage" indicating the peeling away of various layers of information and meaning. Dick Higgins and his "Something Else Press" published works by most of the artists associated with Fluxus and Happenings: George Brecht, John Cage, Allan Kaprow, Alison Knowles, Dick Higgins, Claes Oldenburg, and two books by Roth. Nurtured by the Conceptual movement of the 1960s and 1970s – the pursuit of anti-object, antimuseum options for artistic endeavors – the page soon became another alternative space, as well as a form for the documentation and communication of the ephemeral works of such Conceptual and Minimal artists as Robert Barry, Agnes Denes, Sol LeWitt, and Lawrence Weiner, to name but a few.

Bookworks continue to proliferate as an established form now subject to the art world's current pluralism and stylistic whims, facing its destiny as editions age and values increase. And still, they have never been defined.

> I might say there have been many attempts to define artists' books, and most would concede that it is difficult to do. For me, artists' books combine poetic, conceptual and visual characteristics. And those are exactly the characteristics of Dieter's work. So it is not surprising that he is the father, the son, and the holy ghost of contemporary artists' books.[9]

Ira Wool's enthusiasm is well founded and he is committed to the pursuit of a quality collection of artists' books – his teacher and guide having been 30 years of bookworks by Roth.

A picture book for children, *kinderbuch,* was Roth's first artists' book, a Swiss Constructivistic work produced in 1954. A typographer and graphic designer, among other trades, Roth tried to manipulate the medium of his livelihood in order to satisfy his creative urgencies.

Roth's *book* of 1958, 1959, and 1964 is a portfolio of 18 to 24 black-and-white or colored sheets with hand-cut slots, unbound for the viewer to browse through, turning the sheets around, changing the order, with each move altering the optical image. In 1964 when Roth taught at Yale, resident artist Josef Albers was impressed with Roth's portfolio/book and offered to trade a painting for one of these works. But when Albers came to Roth's studio to pick up his copy (Roth was not there at the time), Albers saw that it was not bound, and would not be. Albers refused to accept an unbound book, exclaiming that the master must decide the whole entity, unable to accept Roth's own conceptual intentions.

Dieter Roth's early works extend from pure, optical, abstract constructions and concrete poetry into experiments with the already-printed page – Icelandic newspapers, comic books, and children's books are bound into editioned volumes with random, unmanipulated sheets or Swiss-cheese-like, die-cut holes, or cut up further and bound to form the miniature *daily mirror* book (1961), a two-centimeter cube. Chopped up books and periodicals also ended up in a sausage skin, mixed with lard, gelatin, and spices in three editions of *Literaturwurst* (1961-70). Food for thought? Indeed. The book is now metamorphosed into another object, each slice a different chapter.

While teaching at the Rhode Island School of Design, Roth wrote the original poems for *scheisse,* the first artists' book in his series of works with this theme and title – books which combine literature and visual art. Roth feels that within whatever categories define his books (pure visual art, pure literature, or a combination of the two), there are subdivisions that must be considered. There are books that try to be good (concrete poetry) and books that try to be bad (*scheisse*). Within these existential subcategories, there are books that succeed or fail intentionally, or not intentionally – in the good sense or in the bad. Roth claims that he used the "scheisse" ("shit") theme to be safe: "...I put it into a shit book so that nobody can blame me – for not having seen it as shit!"[10] Typographical errors made by the students at the Rhode Island School of Design who were unfamiliar with the German language altered the *scheisse* poetry. Does that mean that Roth succeeded or failed in creating *scheisse*? Roth's comment on the students' contributions exacerbates the question with his own relentless self-analysis: "Was good for *scheisse*, but only for the planned *scheisse* – I never could get any real *scheisse*."[11]

Roth continued his quest for real "scheisse," revising the original work into new works, fragmenting and digesting those into a total excretion of ten volumes, the earlier editions almost totally lost in the ultimate, violent self-absorption. One staple through the middle of 112 sheets of text, drawings, photographs, collages, and reliefs affixes these contents to the cover of *(copley book),* a collaborative work between Roth and Richard Hamilton. Roth was introduced to Hamilton by Daniel Spoerri and Jean Tinguely in 1961. Although

Hamilton's subtle, cerebral approach and calculated execution would appear antithetical to impulsive, messy Roth, the two have shared conceptual and literal interests over the years. Hamilton, who served as the printing supervisor on this project (the result of Roth's 1960 award from the William and Noma Copley Foundation in Chicago), produced the book from five years of correspondence and written instructions from Roth, his interpretations and interjections adding one more level of meaning to this difficult, indirect work.

In *MUNDUNCULUM* (1967) the image of a rubber stamp grows into new forms from an invented alphabet of 23 rubber-stamp characters. And if you wish to create your own images, just open up the accompanying *Stemplekasten* (rubber stamp box): Inside, there await twelve rubber stamps from *MUNDUNCULUM,* two stamp pads, and two bottles of ink.

A series of farcical essays (1971-72) were originally conceived as the second part of *MUNDUNCULUM.* In *2 PROBLEME UNSERER ZEIT* (*2 PROBLEMS OF OUR TIME*), Roth filled each page with columns repeating one word, the entire book together forming a single ludicrous sentence; in *ÜBER DAS VERHALTEN DES ALLGEMEINEN ZU ODER GEGENÜBER DEM BESONDEREN BEZIEHUNGSWEISE DES BESONDEREN ZU ORDER GEGENÜBER DEM ALLGEMEINEN* (*ON THE RELATION OF THE GENERAL TO ORDER A SPECIAL OR THE GENERAL ORDERING A SPECIAL I.E. THE SPECIAL ORDERING A GENERAL*) words are merged, the letters extending the sentence continuously through the pages of the book.

Die Tränenmeere und ihre Verwandten (*The Seas of Tears and their Relatives*) is the title of a group of artists' books that originated with Roth's purchase of space in Lucerne's *Luzerner Stadtanzeiger* newspaper two times per week for one and one-half years (beginning in 1971) for the purpose of publishing a series of silly, nonsensical, grammatically improper German sentences. Located on the left-hand page and set off by a rectangle and Roth's initials, these sentences progressively grew more serious and sentimental – a sentence like "Somebody who serves me two steaks will get one steak back from me," leads to "Where does time stay? It stays where it goes away."[12] The newspaper staff, with one and one-half years of this material in hand, stopped the project after one year, having read what was to come. But that did not stop Roth from continuing on his path. In 1973 he published *der Tränensee* (*the Lake of Tears*), an edition of 1200-page bound volumes of these newspapers; *Das TRÄNENMEER* (*The SEA OF TEARS*) volume one, each sentence now isolated on the front of each page, continuing to *Das TRÄNENMEER* volume two's coupling of each of these sentences with a drawing on the preceding page. *Dars Wähnen* (*Ther Vaining*) (1974), volume three of *The SEA OF TEARS,* places the drawings from volume two opposite a new text that now deals with the image from a new point of view. This contextually referential, self-conscious series continues in the fourth volume, *Das Weinen* (*Crying*) (1978), which is also volume 2A of *Das Wähnen,* the text now extended to a theatrical play.

Dieter Roth's *Collection of Flat Waste* gives us a version of Roth's diary in the direct, specific, digested sense, as he slips all of his collected flat or flattened waste into the plastic sleeves of a binder for us to flip through, greeting this man by browsing through his garbage. An early collection, retained from 1975-76, consists of Roth's daily debris from one year, a 365-volume set, whereas one week of this practice in 1982 delivers thirty-one volumes of translucent sleeves, slowly revealing and dissolving the numerous cigarette butts, film wrappers, and even a letter from Ira Wool in this compulsive, self-analytic work (fig. 4).

Dieter Roth's *Collected Works* are offset volumes of republished and previously unpublished works, reproduced as is or in a manipulated state, with exotic, deluxe-edition covers collaging everything from plastic turds to smashed light bulbs swimming in glue, to a collaborative cassette tape with Fluxus video artists Nam June Paik and Charlotte Moorman. Of approximately 80 of these collected works, Roth has managed to publish 23: consecutive through volume 20, but not chronological with regard to the original works, the numbers then jump to volume 36, 40, and then to 38, as Roth produces work which only superficially alludes to order; there is no straightening out of the spiral tower. Volumes 20, 40, and 38 deal specifically with this issue: Although catalogues of his books and graphics from 1947 to 1980, these works offer order in presentation only. The impeccable attention to detail, Hansjörg Mayer's systematic precision in reproductive and typographical uniformity and scale, and the clinically detailed cataloguing of each book and graphic, are deceptive in their application to the real products. The apparent approachability of these clean, bi-lingual volumes only skims the surface of these works, as if to fool those who can deal only with order and appearance before they can deal with substance and concept. The real entity is not an anchor in time, and not a predigested map of Roth's spiral tower. For the sake of apparent order, chronology takes precedence, breaking up sequences, styles, and series. The compulsive consistency in the reduced reproduction is even applied to the minute *daily mirror* book. Roth shows us that you cannot judge his books by their covers (or even from a hint of what is inside) or by a menu of ingredients. These purely printed catalogues remain static, contained by the deceptive presentation, as the editions are dispersed and the organics die. The spiral remains in anarchy.

Dieter Roth's graphic work is grounded in his training in typography and design. Again, there are collaborations, including a number of joint efforts with Stephen Wewerka. Roth's imagination and emotions stretch the boundaries of this medium to let the world seep in. Intaglio, lithography, woodcuts, and serigraphy are all in use, often at the same time; fluctuations in the final edition are the result of added painting and drawing or the exotic materials that he presses between the plate and paper. Roth's pictorial expressions include numerous self-portraits (as dogs, clouds, air, etc.), images within images, heads within heads – surrealistically composed – like the self-conscious *Christa* (fig. 5), the "American Female Christ."[13]

As with every technology and medium that Dieter Roth employs, redefinition metabolizes to de-definition. Graphics are no longer conventional flat, static, multiple images – though Roth takes advantage of the salability of such works. What appear to be unique paintings and sculpture are actually multiples: A cast chocolate-covered board supports the frozen images of three motorcyclists, as the object dehydrates in real time (fig. 6); thirty-six chocolate wafers and curdled milk are sealed between two pieces of plastic, with the subsequent molding a by-product obscuring the image (fig. 7); and two small rabbit figurines (fig. 8) on closer inspection are molded rabbit droppings, earth, and straw, made in the same device that turns out the edible chocolate editions at Easter.

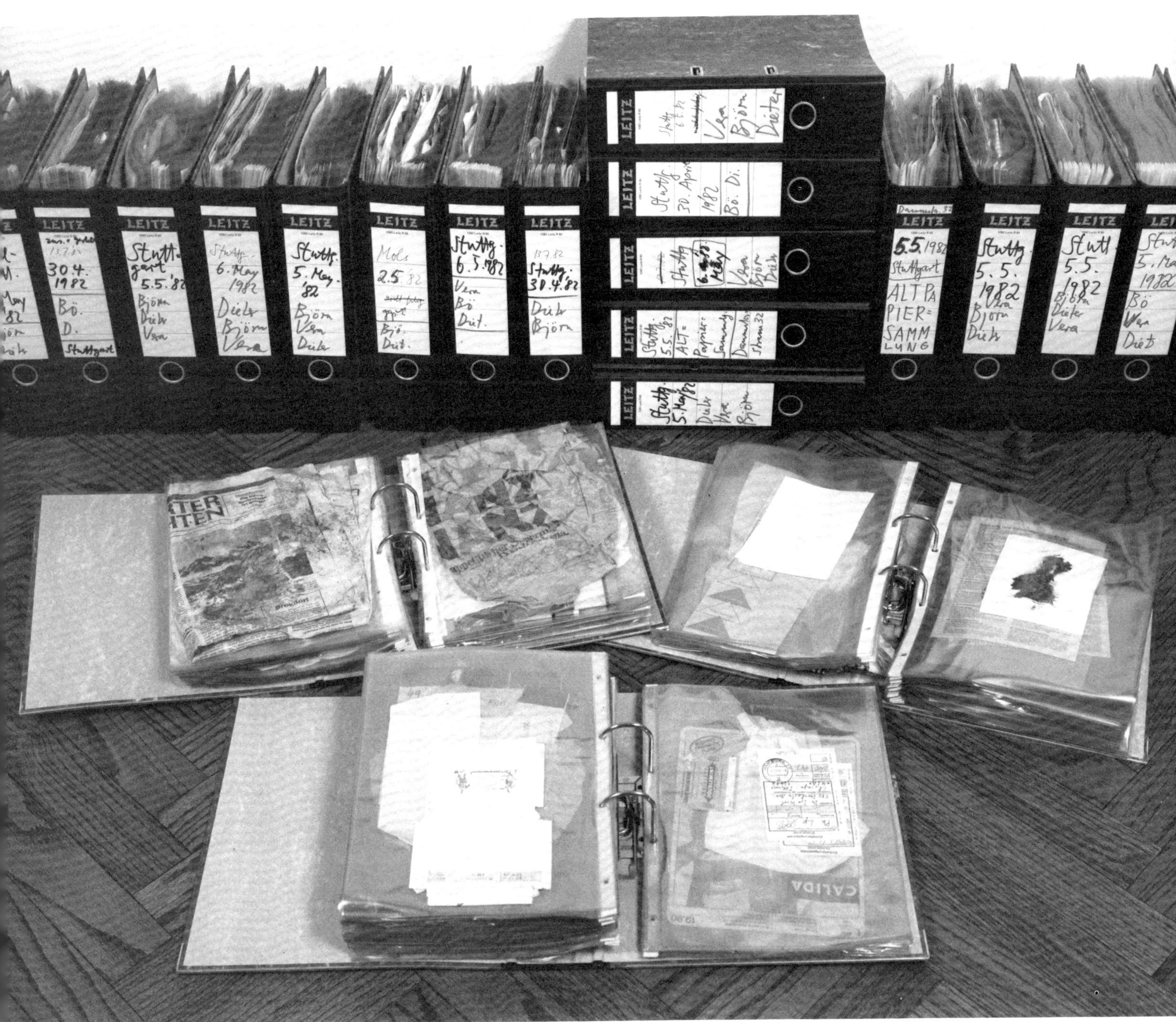

Fig. 4.
Sammlung flachen Abfalls 1982 (Collection of Flat Waste 1982), 1982. Printed matter, packages, notes, labels, etc. in files, each piece in a transparent folder.

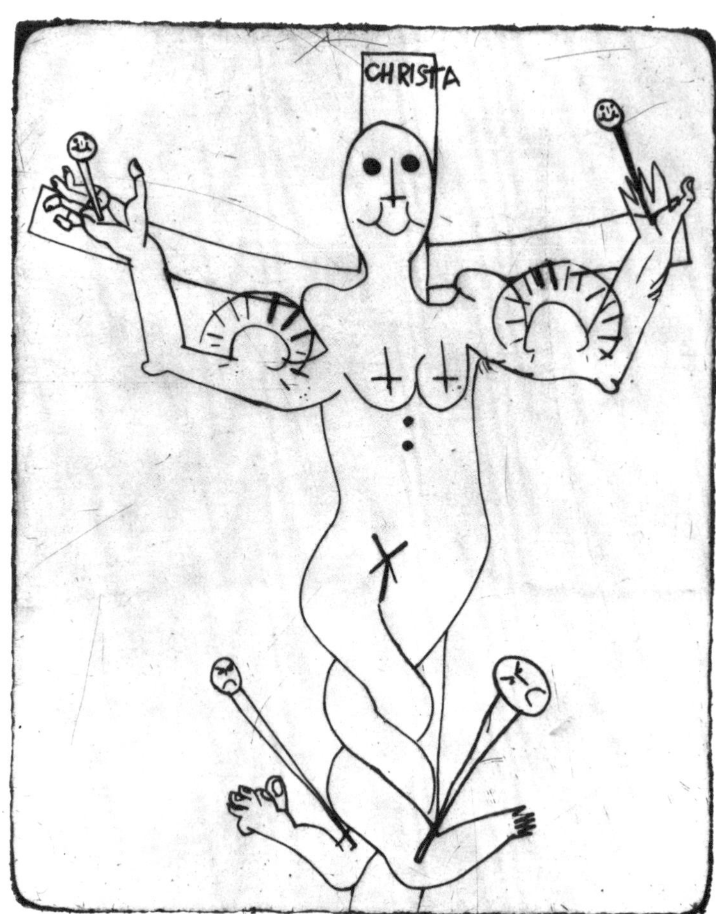

Fig. 5.
Christa, 1966. Etching.

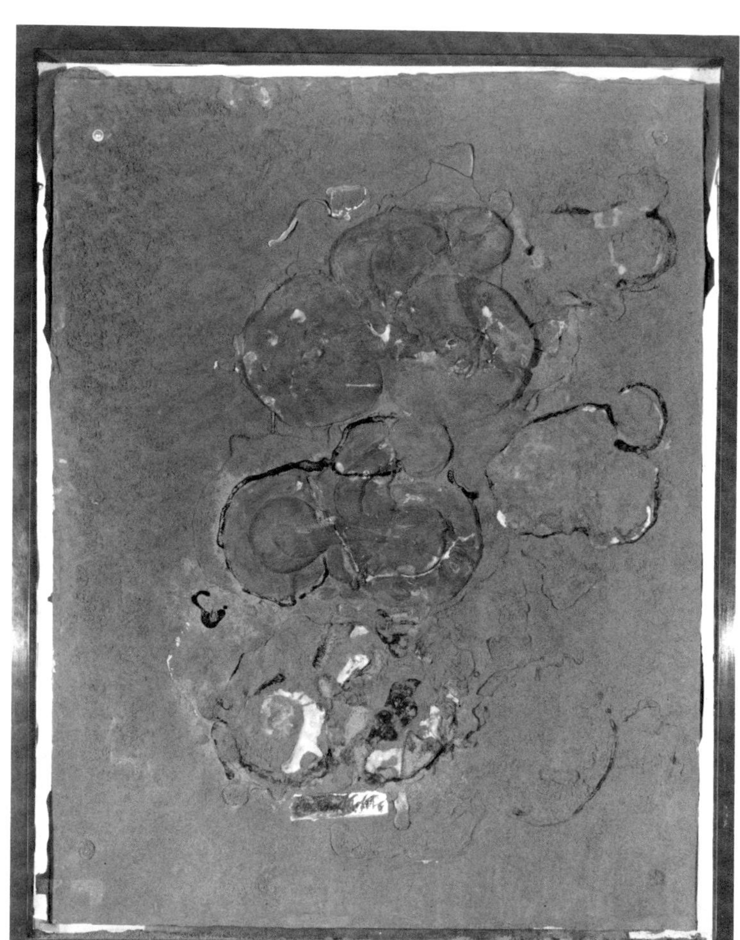

Fig. 6.
Motorradfahrerungoüch (Motorcycle driver's misfortune), 1976-77. Chocolate on board with glue, bolts, and washers.

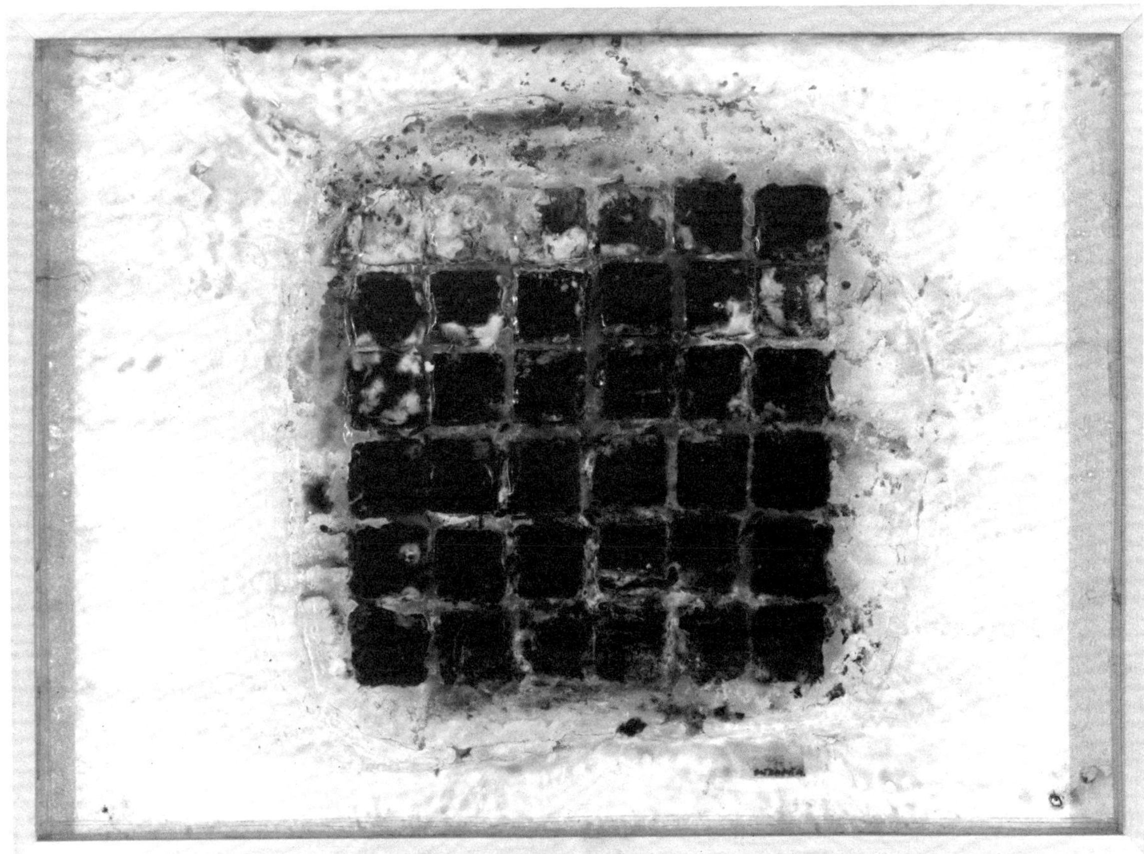

Fig. 7.
chocoladenpoätzchenbild (chocolatewafer picture), 1969. Filled chocolate wafers and curdled milk in plastic cover.

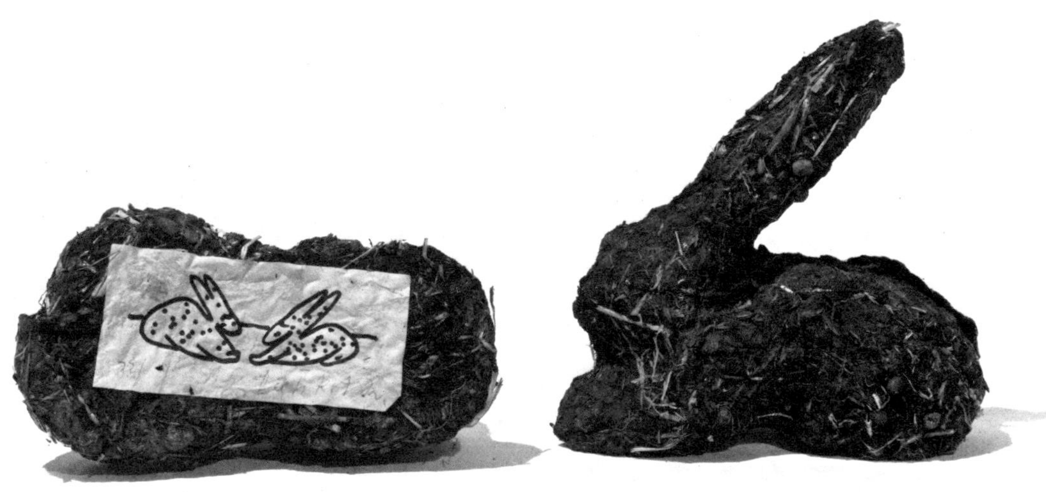

Fig. 8.
Untitled (two rabbits), 1975. Earth, straw, and rabbit droppings.

Roth is not alone in his use of food and the organic in graphics and multiples. Another prime example is American artist Edward Ruscha, who shares with Roth a commerical art background and a preoccupation with the printed word and the production of artists' books. Ruscha has used everything from chocolate to caviar, baked beans, squid, and red-currant jelly as a printing medium (for example, in his series "News," "Mews," "Pews," "Brews," "Stews," "Dues," in 1970). Still, despite the similarity of process, these two artists produce very different work: Roth's intensely messy, heaving, existential approach to food cannot be compared to Ruscha's subtle, refined handling of these materials; indeed, Ruscha experiments with the organic palette, excluding those materials which would mold.

At the XXXV Venice Biennale in 1970 Edward Ruscha installed his *Chocolate Room* – 360 sheets printed with chocolate through open silkscreens and hung on the wall like chocolate shingles; the surfaces were altered by wetted fingertips and a population of ants. The same year, at the Eugenia Butler Gallery in Los Angeles, Roth installed 40 suitcases filled with a variety of cheeses and called it *Staple Cheese, a Race.* Roth recalled:

> There's a saying in German that goes: "Who's left this suitcase here?" and is used when people break wind. I decided to create works of art about this saying.
>
> I had a show of 40 suitcases, large, small, old and new, and all of them were full of cheese. There were two tons of cheese in that show. It was like a train terminal, suitcases everywhere. The people in Los Angeles didn't know the German saying but they noticed the smell. There was a heatwave on the West Coast at the time. In a few days the suitcases had begun to leak, there were pools on the floor and the smell indescribable. A cloud formed over the city. Soon flies and insects started to arrive and the gallery was covered with flies. The lady who owned the gallery sat there for six hours everyday and couldn't see anything because of the flies, although both the walls and the floor were originally painted white. Eventually there were so many flies about that you couldn't get through the gallery. They were so dazed by the smell of the cheese that they covered the walls like thick paint. Then the police came, investigated this fly-business and said: Close the gallery. The gallery-owner's husband was a lawyer and he said: We stay open. There was a lot of fuss. Sanitary inspectors were brought in and they found that the cheese had formed vapours akin to laughing gas, which could be dangerous. Then the gallery lady, who'd sat in the place for six hours everyday, said: I was wondering why I felt so merry the whole time.[14]

This year of food art also included Daniel Spoerri's *Homage to Diter Rot,* an old-fashioned stove with bread bursting out of the doors, burners, and pots. Indeed, other artists, too, were experimenting with the use of food: Joseph Beuys in Düsseldorf and the Nouveaux Réalistes in Paris had been employing the organic in their work. This exploration of the conceptual and emotive possibilities of unconventional materials has continued into present-day performances and installations by these and many other artists. In his own experimentation, however, Roth has always moved on:

> It's important to exhibit your mistakes. Man is not perfect, neither are his creations. I've given up using sour milk. Instead I use music. I sometimes

> fasten a tape recorder onto paintings or objects and have the music pour over the spectator/listener. This creates a certain effect: Those who look at the art don't realize how bad it is when they hear the music. For the music is even worse. Two bad things make one good thing.[15]

Roth's ideas toward music can be traced back to neo-Dada Fluxus origins, the incorporations of everyday life, chance, and randomness in the music and scores of John Cage, George Brecht, Dick Higgins, Yoko Ono, and others, as well as to the cacaphonous "rarely heard music" symphonies – collaborations with Austrian Actionists Hermann Nitsch, Oswald Wiener, Günter Brus, and others.

In 1982 Roth installed two musical works in the Galerie Bama in Paris. One, a work from 1978, was itself a sequel to Roth's collaboration with Richard Hamilton which involved an exhibition for dogs – dog-interest images of sausages, other dogs, etc., with a manipulated Don Quixote theme hung at dog height. Roth was later told of a restaurant in Barcelona that supplied a special menu for dogs. He recalled:

> I went there. I asked for the Dog-menu which proved to be both exquisite and expensive. I asked the waiter why they had a special menu for

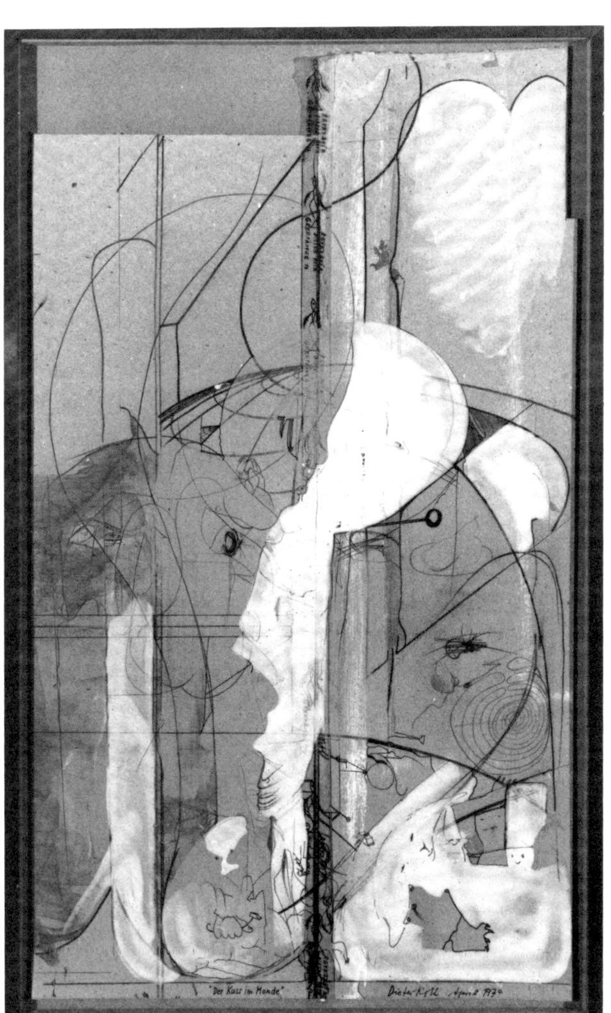

Fig. 9.
Der Kuss im Monde (The Kiss in the Moon), 1974. Paint, glue, pencil, ink, and cellophane tape on board.

> dogs and why the prices were so high. He led me out on the balcony and asked me to listen carefully, and I heard emerging from the darkness the painful howl of dogs. The music moved me so profoundly so I asked the waiter about the connection between it and the menu. "We donate the income from the Dog-menu to a Retreat for dogs that people have abandoned.... The dogpeople become so depressed, so melancholic, that they die in a week or two. But before they die they complain about their maltreatment by howling like this."[16]

Roth immediately made a tape recording of 24 hours of this "dog music." He filled albums with 2000 self-portraits as a dog and 1400 photographs of the dogs at the Retreat, and installed the lot in a show in Madrid. He also set up equipment to record all of the current sounds within the gallery and offices. The recordings from Madrid were taken to a Swiss exhibition and dubbed by Roth with Swiss babble.

Roth's second installation at Galerie Bama, in 1982, *Musical tableaux objects,* filled one room with tape recorders which played and recorded continuously as spectators participated and added sounds to the piece by typing at a typewriter and playing the electric organ. Roth stretched the boundaries of each medium through his pursuit of real-life, real-time reactions.

Dieter Roth's paintings and drawings continue his autobiographical, lyrical wanderings. Here, too, his lively, vivid, dialectical expressions and use of the organic and unconventional pass through the styles, stages, and materials of the bookworks, bypassing intimacy for direct confrontation: early design-oriented paintings, paintings formed primarily of glue (see fig. 9) or of chocolate, palettes that have become paintings (see fig. 10), rubberbands stretched around an Uecker-like nailed surface (fig. 11), other paintings as underpaintings, a multitude of self-portraits, or simply a line drawing on the reverse of a paper placemat of two heads engulfing each other, entitled *2 Cannibals* (fig. 12); or, as

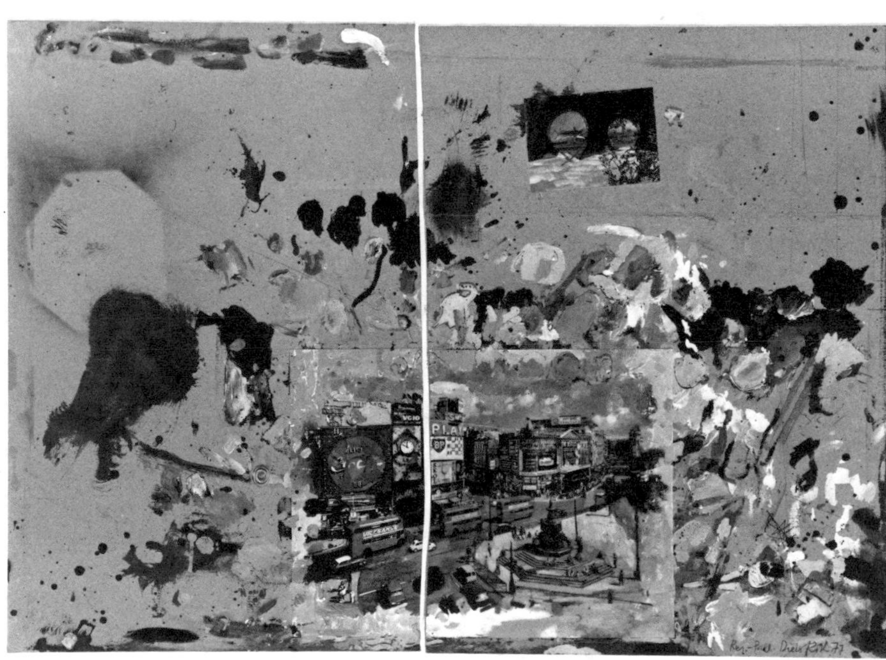

Fig. 10.
Untitled (Piccadilly Palette Painting), 1977. Paint, paint tube, glue, glue tube, plastic marker top, pencil, offset postcard, and offset (Piccadilly) print on two boards mounted on masonite.

Fig. 11.
gummibandbild (rubberband painting), 1981.
Nails, wood, black paint, and rubberbands.

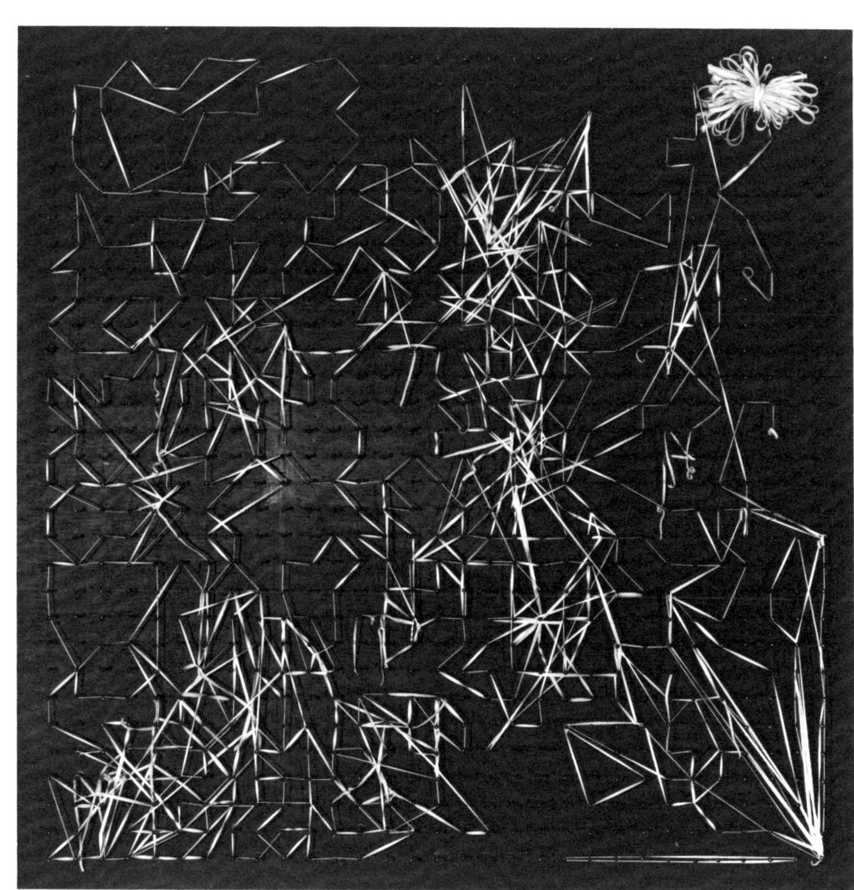

Fig. 12.
2 Cannibals, 1977. Ink with food stains on placemat from The Parthenon, Chicago.

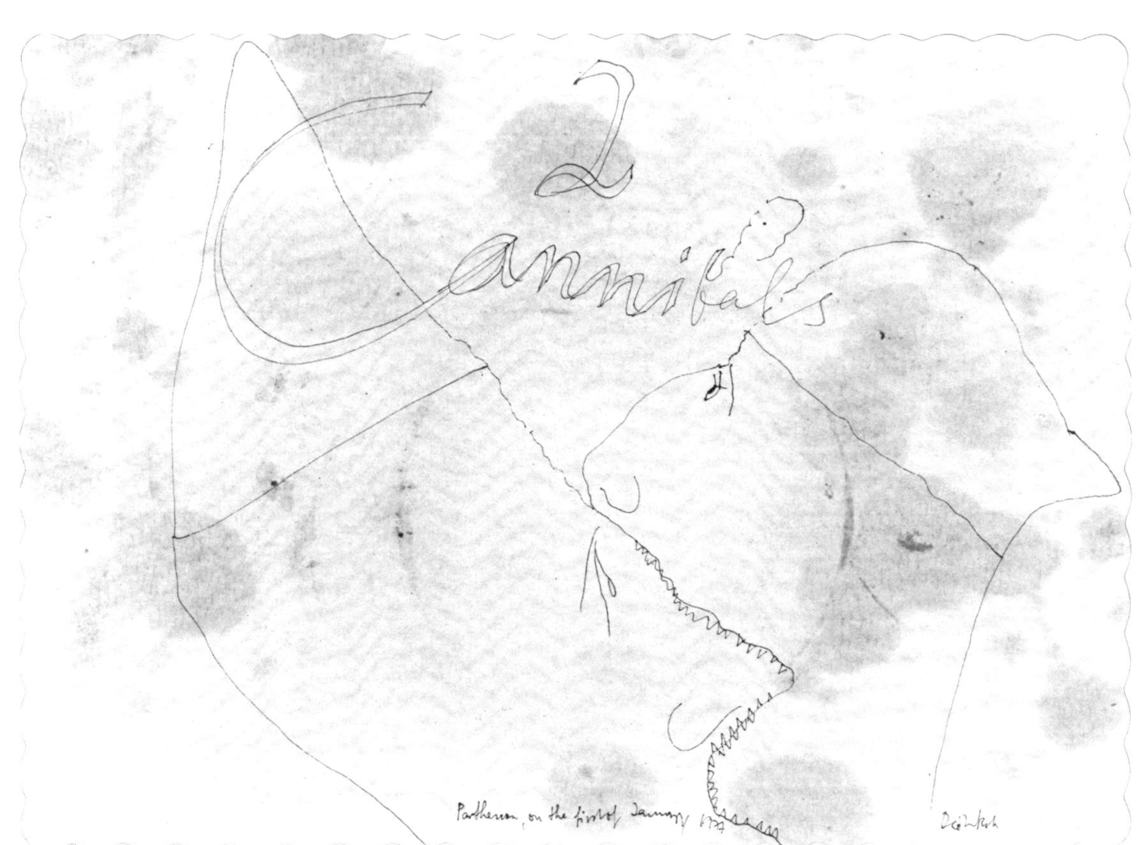

in *Chicago Wandbild*, the transformation of Ira Wool's kitchen wall into a multimedia extravaganza, perhaps the culmination of this collaborative friendship. Wool recalled:

> I had talked to Dieter a number of times about coming to Chicago. He told me one day that he had this idea that he would like to go around repainting each year all the paintings he had done, and so we talked about him coming to Chicago and repainting paintings as one possibility. Then he thought about painting the windowshades, so that in the winter you could pull down the shades and have a summer scene, or something of that order. He also talked about painting a mural, which didn't appeal to me because I wasn't sure how long I was going to live in that apartment and obviously I couldn't take the mural with me.
>
> By the time he came, in 1976, he decided that what he'd do was make the mural on panels which he could attach to the wall. We went to an art supply store and bought the canvases – I believe there were four of them to start with, each three-by-four feet – and he would always work on them in the guest bedroom, two at a time. Dieter was going to teach me how to paint, and actually there are some strokes somewhere under there on those panels which I made. He told me the most important thing in painting was learning how to wash the brushes, but not very much on how to use them.
>
> Over the years the mural's just grown until it has filled one entire wall. It even has a sound track, with tape loops made by Dieter, and some with Dieter and his children, singing or playing music, on standard instruments like piano or cello, or on dimestore instruments. The idea is that the painting is going to have speakers, and that each of the painted figures on the panels will have a voice.
>
> ...One time when Dieter was here he prepared us a meal, and the menu for that meal is in the painting. There are postcards from him in other places. It's a work which is always commenting on itself.
>
> ...Another thing is, I consider it his. I have the work on my wall, it stays here, but it belongs to Dieter.[17]

Just as the *Chicago Wandbild* can in part be considered a collaborative work, springing from Roth's personal relationship with the Wools, so Roth has frequently been involved in more direct collaborations with other artists.

Roth and Richard Hamilton fused their individual identities into the collective "Ch. Rotham" for their 1976 "Collaborations" exhibition of co-produced works (paintings, drawings, prints, and writings) done in Cadaqués, Spain, during a three-week period just prior to the installation. Hamilton had prepared many of the works prior to his arrival, his labored efforts immediately transformed by Roth. Anticipating questions regarding the true authorship and authenticity of each of these collaborative works, Roth and Hamilton produced "certificates" for each piece; for example, for *Replica of "Portrait of the Artist by Francis Bacon by Dieter Roth"* (fig. 13) the "certificate" (fig. 14) is a drawing of this painting which itself is based on a 1970 image by Richard Hamilton made from a Polaroid taken of Bacon by Hamilton. The certificate is complete with a signed and witnessed statement of dubious authenticity written in deconstructive language that turns the whole effort back onto itself. Roth and

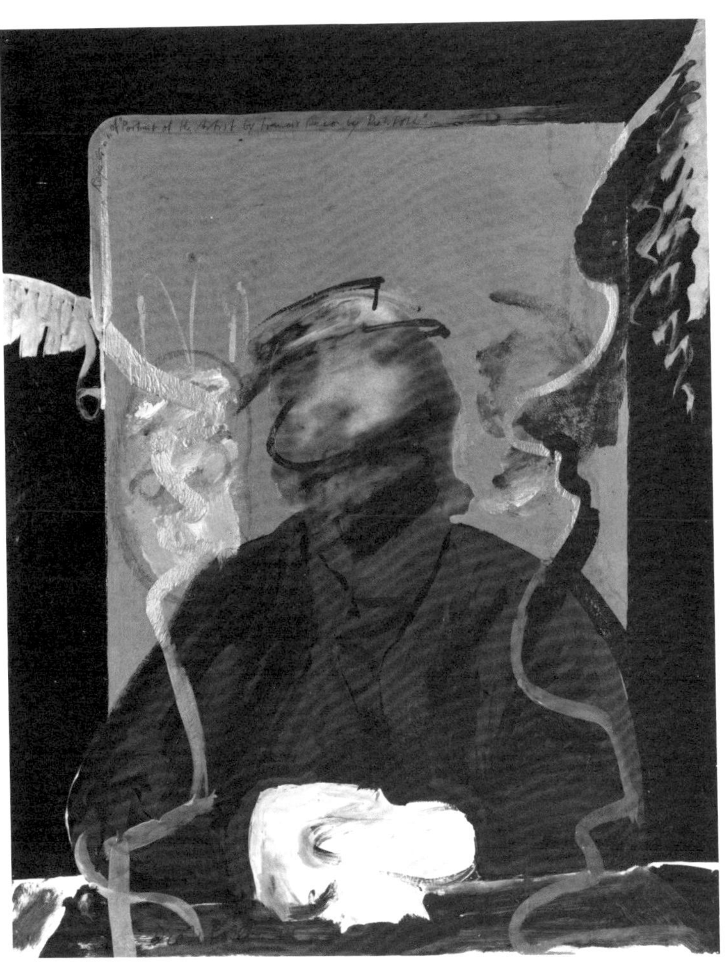

Fig. 13.
Replica of "Portrait of the Artist by Francis Bacon by Dieter Roth," 1976.
Paint on paper.

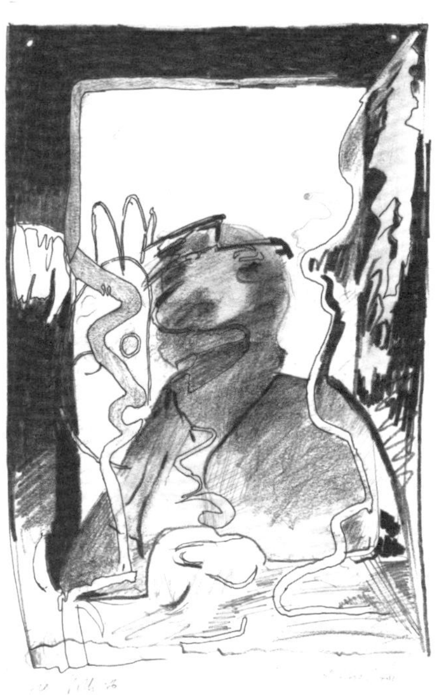

Fig. 14.
Dieter Roth/Richard Hamilton.
Certificate for Replica of "Portrait of the artist by Fr. B. by D.R.," 1976.
8 B Faber-Castell pencil and Rotring ink on handmade paper.

Hamilton set us up for confusion, and ensure it by covering all paths to solution.

Austrian artist Arnulf Rainer shares Roth's preoccupation with the self. Rainer's recent graphically manipulated photographs transform, exaggerate, and maim his photographic body. Although Rainer's performances are confined to the privacy of the studio, he is a contemporary of the Vienna Actionists, known for their public performances dating back to the 1960s, the sadomasochistic acts of ritual disembowelment of animals, public defecation, and self-mutilation. These works by Hermann Nitsch, Günter Brus, Otto Mühl, the late Rudolf Schwarzkogler, Valie Export, and others have been performed for the purposes of socio-political, personal, and fantastic catharsis.

Together, Roth and Rainer formed "Misch- u. Trennkunst" (Mix and Divi Art), a cooperative firm established in 1973. They have collaborated on video, audio, and photographic projects: a confrontation of two deeply self-analytic personalities, a dynamic encounter, Roth's lyricism and burlesque humor offsetting Rainer's hysterical contortions, as both artists are caught up in the theatrics of it all (see fig. 15).

What Roth does not invent he transforms. Postcards and letters to the Wools, painted images of people or monsters, were once offset images of Chicago's Ba'hai Temple, Wrigley Field, or Icelandic women in national costumes. Roth claims this mode of correspondence is easier than writing a letter.

Velázquez's mirror-image *Las Meninas* is "mirrored" again by Roth, who cuts two identical postcards of this image and replaces the top above the top and the bottom below the bottom, repainting the mismatched half to reunify the image (fig. 16).

The vibrating scene of London's Piccadilly Circus, with its interacting components, the bright red Coca-Cola sign, the statue of Eros, and the parade of double-decker buses, is the subject of 96 alterations and manipulations – an image in flux (fig. 17). Published also in book form as volume 36 of the *Collected Works,* it includes Roth's Joycean foreword, a diatribe that disintegrates through repetitions. In turn, the cards themselves are delineated so as to be cut out of the book and dispersed. Roth additionally extends this image through prints, as well as the deluxe-edition bookcover: an original double Piccadilly painting over the double offset print of the postcard image (fig. 18).

Many artists have extended letters into drawings and paintings, for example, Jean Tinguely and H. C. Westermann. Roth's wide range of erratic styles and temperaments jumps through his letters. His style wanders, as the pictorial continues the self-analytic, self-deprecating humor, now on a personalized level (see fig. 19), while the thousands of books, filled with excerpts from diaries and intimate images, are sent into the artistic diaspora, for strangers to share.

Whereas many artists concern themselves with perfection and reception of their precious products which are distinct from the products of the everyday encounter, Roth is preoccupied with bringing life back into his art. The trail of works that Dieter Roth casts into the world reveals an oeuvre that is not so much linear as horizontally dynamic. One piece reacts to the next, each layered with distractions and obstacles to the meaning – which remains with Roth. It is surprising that this passionate individualist, constrained by a basic fear of people, delights in and often initiates collaborations with other artists. The play of styles, the merging, submerging, and confrontations of personalities in these encounters continue the hybridization of Dieter Roth's art.

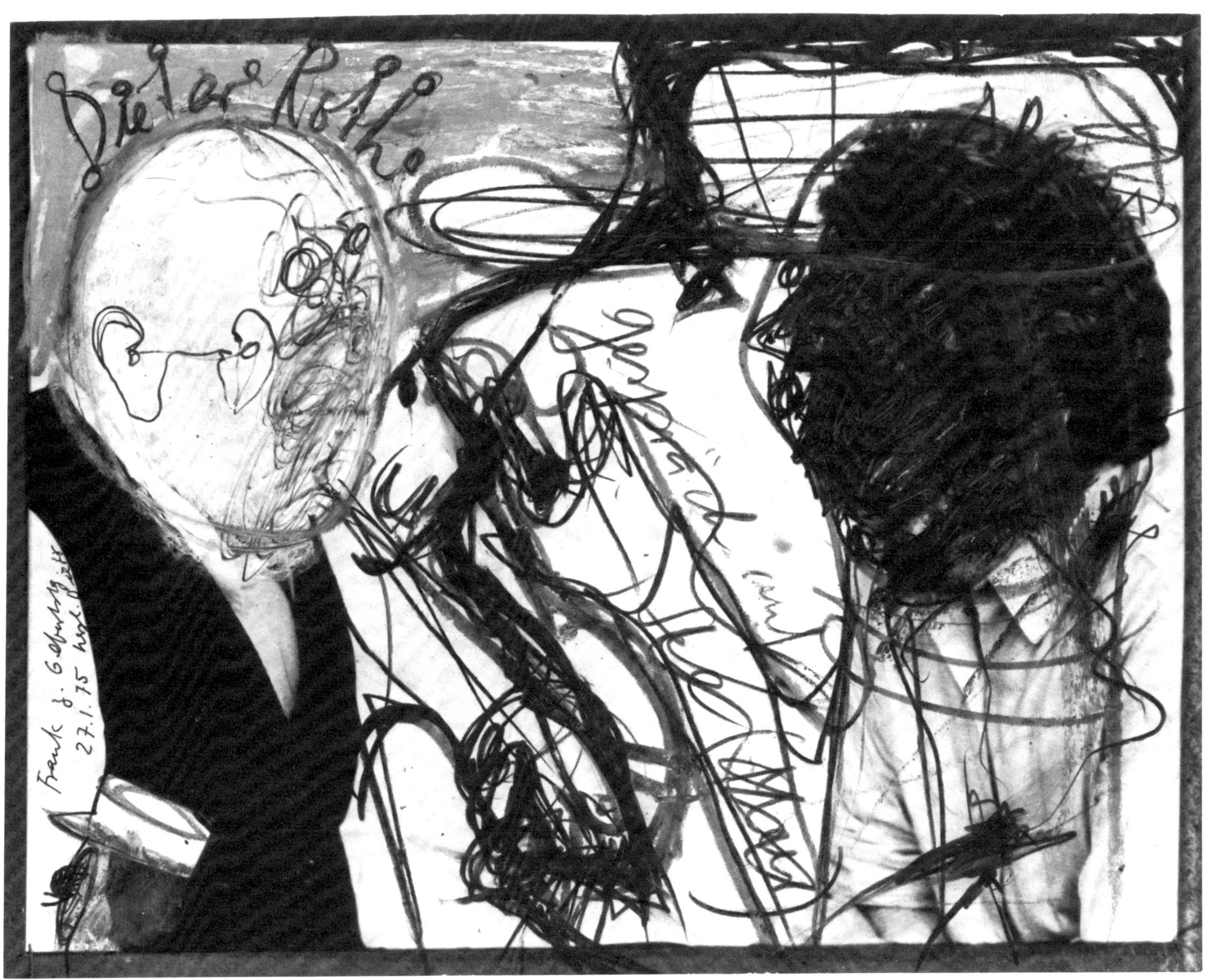

Fig. 15.
Gespräch (Dialogue), 1975. Oil pastel and pencil on photograph.

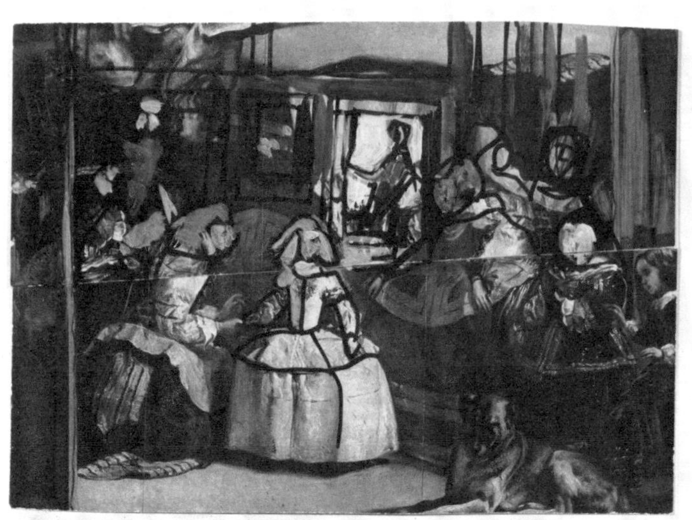

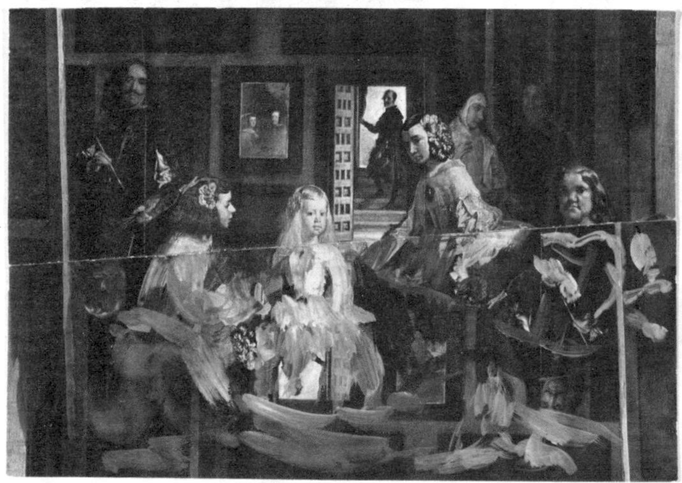

Fig. 16.
Las Meninas (from the "Cloisters Series"), 1977.
Paint and felt-tip pen on postcards.

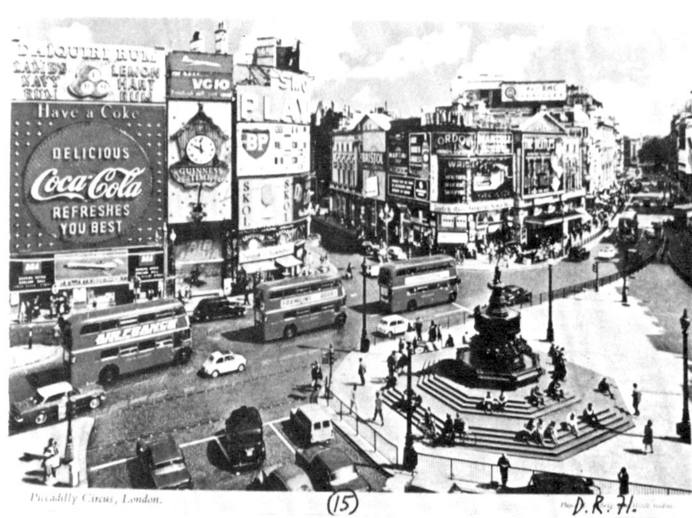

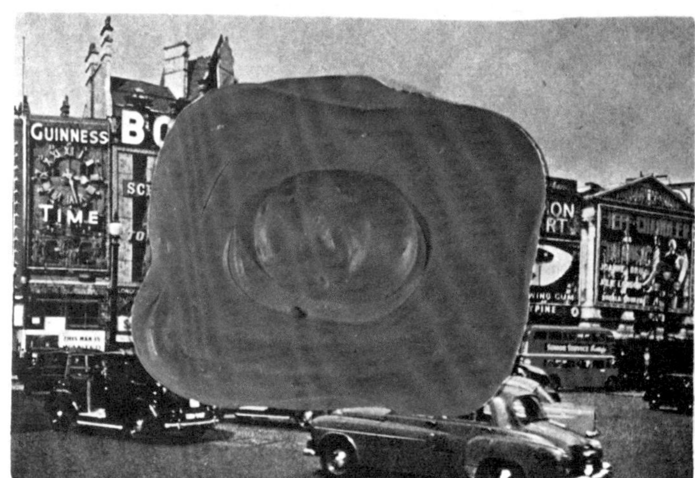

Fig. 17.
96 Piccadillies (Stuttgart-London: Edition Hansjörg Mayer, 1977).
Top: "1/Piccadilly Circus, London (ca. 1965)/Picture Postcard from a suite of 16, 1971"; Bottom: "2/Postcard to Rita Donagh, 1968/Acrylic on offset printing on card." Collection of Museum of Contemporary Art, Chicago.

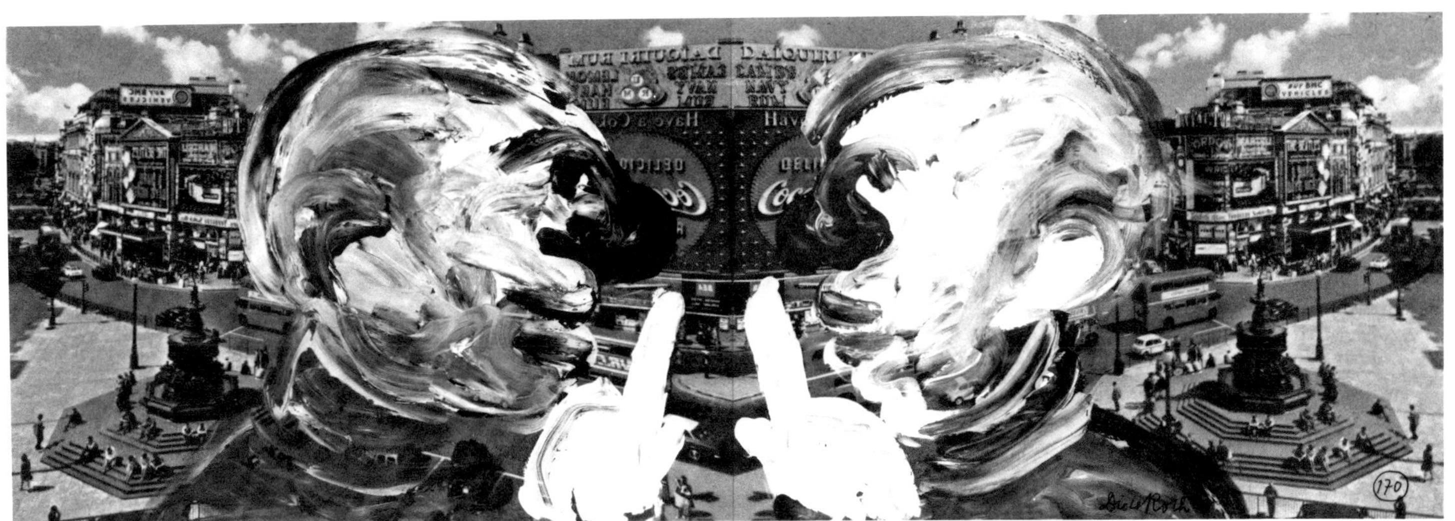

Fig. 18.
Doublepiccadilly Painting, 1979. Paint on offset print.

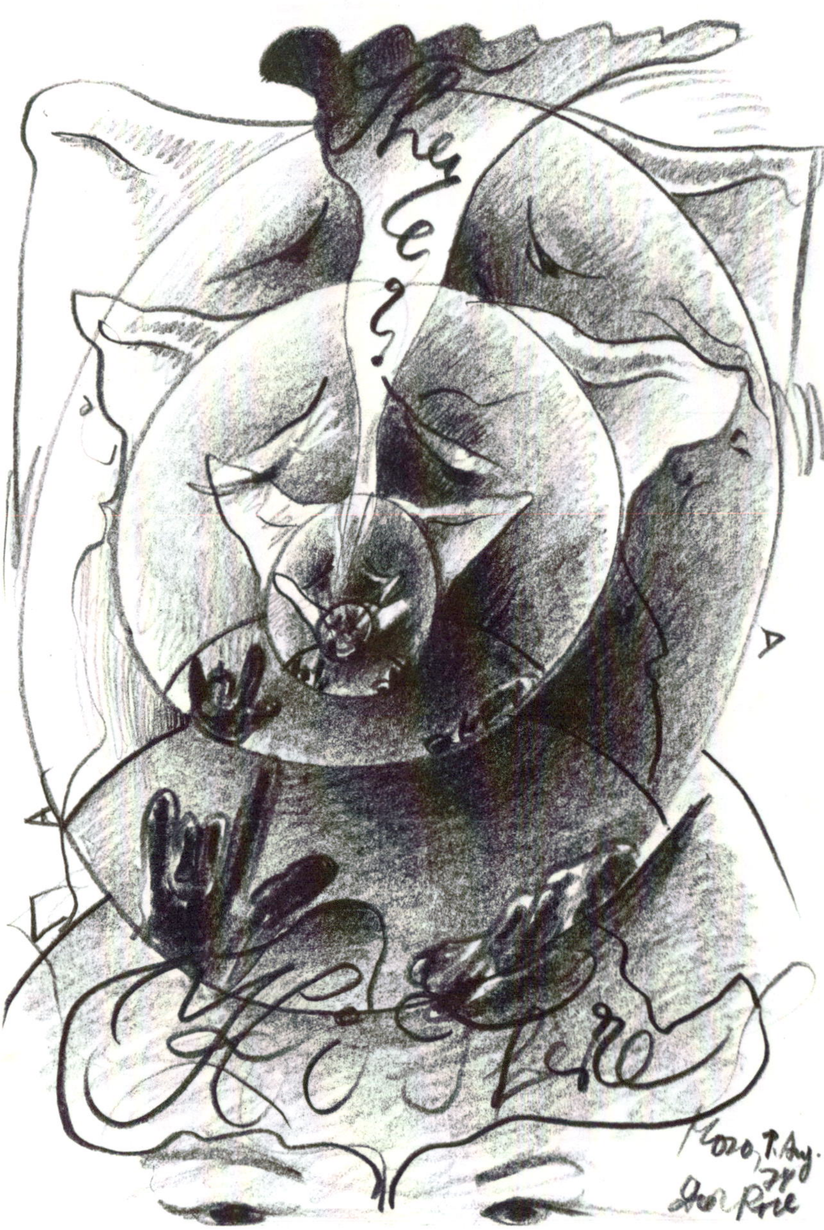

Fig. 19.
Untitled (Hi There), 1978. Pencil on paper.

Notes

1. Buzz Spector, "Interview with Ira Wool," *The Flue* (Franklin Furnace, New York) (Winter 1983): 13.

2. Ibid.

3. Dieter Roth in Richard Hamilton and Dieter Roth, *Collaborations of Ch. Rotham* (Stuttgart: Edition Hansjörg Mayer, and Cadaqués [Gerona], Spain: Galeria Cadaqués, 1977): 121.

4. "'I only extract the square root,' Dieter Roth speaks. An Interview by Ingólfur Margeirsson in *Pjóöviljinn,* September 3, 1978," in *Dieter Roth,* exh. cat. Nýlistasafnid – The Living Art Museum, Reykjavík, 1982: 8.

5. Ibid.: 6-7.

6. Ira Wool, "Interview with Dieter Roth," Chicago (Oct. 1978): videotape.

7. John Willett, "Look, No Frontiers," *Studio International* 183, 941 (Feb. 1972): 49.

8. Dieter Schwarz, Introduction to *96 Piccadillies,* vol. 36 in *Collected Works* by Dieter Roth (London: Eaton House, 1977): 136. The author is indebted to Dieter Schwarz for his extensive material available in English on the work of Dieter Roth. It has proved invaluable in the interpretation of Roth's German-language works as well as for an initial chronology of Roth's name. For a catalogue raisonné of Roth's works up to 1981, and an extensive bibliography, see Dieter Schwarz, *AUF DER BOGEN BAHN*... (Zurich: Seedorn Verlag, 1981).

9. Spector (note 1): 13.

10. Wool (note 6).

11. Ibid.

12. Ibid.

13. Ibid.

14. "I only extract the square root" (note 4): 8-9.

15. Ibid.: 8.

16. Ari Kristinsson and Eggert Einarsson, "From an Essay on Dieter Roth" (1978) in *Dieter Roth,* exh. cat. Nýlistasafnid – The Living Art Museum, Reykjavík, 1982: 11.

17. Spector (note 1): 19.